Paleo Diet Challenge

Beginner's Guide To Rapid Weight Loss And Unlimited Energy

(30 Day Paleo Challenge)

Brandon Ward

TERMS & CONDITIONS

No part of this book should be transmitted or reproduced in any form whatsoever, including electronic, print, scanning, photocopying, recording or mechanical without the prior written permission of the author. All the information, ideas and guidelines are for educational purpose only. The writer has tried to ensure the utmost accuracy of the content provided in the book, all the readers are advised to follow instructions at their own risk. The author of this book cannot be held liable for any incidental damage, personal or even commercial caused by misrepresentation of the information given in the book. Readers are encouraged to seek professional help when needed.

Table of Contents

Chapter 1: What is Paleo Diet & How Does It Work?

The very name "paleo diet" is a shortened version of "Paleolithic diet". Primitive people, who lived in the Paleolithic period, which ended 11000 years ago, did not know what a microwave oven is & didn't eat convenience foods. In that era, agriculture was not yet developed & people practically didn't eat dairy products & cereals. Sugar, bread & other "pleasures" of the modern diet were completely unknown to the ancient man! They were hunters & gathers. Some modern nutritionists call the paleo diet the most natural food system, no matter what century we live in.

This diet consists of trying to return to our beginnings & develop a diet that is based on those foods that cavemen used to eat ages ago. To lose weight, get healthier & be completely transformed, specialists recommend to imitate our ancestors diet. This means that your diet should mainly consist of meat & fish dishes, a considerable amount of vegetables & fruits in fresh form, in addition to nuts, seeds & mushrooms. In reasonable quantities, it is permissible to consume vegetable oils. It is recommended to eliminate legumes, dairy products, fatty meats, cereals, vegetables rich in carbs, & food with high salt content, like convenience foods & salted nuts because salt has negative effect on kidneys & leads to pain in the joints.

The fact is that in the primitive times, it was difficult to survive, so people tried to eat mostly the products that are simply to find & get. Moreover, they constantly small game & hunted birds, which in modern society is easily replaced by physical activity. The main characteristic of paleo diet is that it doesn't impose certain restrictions on the amount of food consumed & on the ways of its preparation, the food you eat is just healthier. Vegetables, fish & meat can be boiled, stewed or fried. It is recommended to prioritize products of organic origin.

The creators of the paleo diet believe that the human digestive system is adapted specifically to food of the Paleolithic period. The human genome has been formed for several million years & those foods that appeared later on are contrary to the biological genetic essence. Our digestive tract, during the course of evolution, has perfectly learned to digest food obtained from hunting &

gathering. For 2.4 million years, mankind didn't drink milk (with the exception of the breastfeeding period) & eat cereals, canned foods, refined & completely went without them.

Agriculture & raising of stock appeared only about 10,050 years ago, which by the standards of the evolutionary processes is like one moment & major changes just could not occur during this time. However, during this time our food has changed dramatically! People have learned to bake bread & grow cereals, cook jam & get sugar, raise livestock, the fat content of which is several times higher than that of their wild relatives. This is not even mentioning all sorts of chemical additives & genetically modified products, the history of which is only a few decades!

Of course, our body cannot keep up with the progress of the food industry, & it is the irrational diet - the consumption of a large number of refined foods, fatty foods, sweets, & obvious overeating, is one of the main reasons for the development of excess weight & a wide range of different diseases. In modern nutrition, this group of products accounts for between fifty & sixty percent of the diet & is the cause of many diseases because at the genetic level, the person doesn't need them. Just bringing your diet back to normal, you may get rid of many health problems.

The adherents of paleo diet believe that the primitive people's diet is most consistent with the human genome, so returning to our origins will allow us to forget about many contemporary diseases & normalize weight. The human body receives the necessary amount of calories from meat. Consuming protein food, remember that it requires physical activity to be digested, which is what our ancestors did while hunting & gathering. Fish contains a large number of polyunsaturated fatty acids, which provide the body with sufficient energy, satisfy hunger & help normalize the concentration of glucose & cholesterol in the blood. The amount of carbs consumed is minimized, so this diet is low-carbohydrate.

Elimination of dairy products & sugar minimizes the likelihood of obesity, & also prevents the development of diabetes. Primitive people, who didn't master agriculture, naturally didn't raise cows, collect milk & prepare the corresponding products. They gave preference to meat, rich in protein & amino acids. Also, milk is not consumed due to the fact that the adult human body doesn't produce enough enzymes for processing lactose, which may be digested only in infancy. It is always recommended to substitute salt with herbs & spices & sweet tea & coffee with plain water (at least 2 quarters should be consumed every day).

Residents of the island of Kitava (Papua New Guinea) are probably the most thoroughly studied settlement of hunter-gatherers & are a great example of the benefits of paleolithic diet in our days. According to physician Staffan Lindeberg, who carefully studied their habits, the Kitavans consume exclusively:

- Fish and seafood
- Coconuts
- Starchy fruits (tapioca, yams, sweet potatoes, taro)
- Vegetables
- Fruits (guava, watermelon, pumpkin, pineapple, mango, banana, papaya)

Kitavans are strong & healthy, they don't have strokes, heart attacks, acne, obesity & diabetes, despite the fact that most of them smoke! They're a great prove that paleo diet is indeed effective.

The Paleo diet is a recreation of the diet of ancient people, but not a repetition of their way of life, as many mistakenly believe. There is no need to independently hunt animals, take a fishing pole & fish or wander through the woods in search of edible roots & berries. All necessary products can be bought from farmers or in specialized organic stores. It's worth noting that this process of eating is not necessarily to be followed only for a short period of time. It may be followed for a long time & slightly adjusted according to personal needs & specifics of the digestive system.

We would really want to believe that there is some kind of inner wisdom that controls our dietary desire, so that we consume the most nutritious food from the point of view of nutrients. However, unfortunately, according to scientific research, in addition to craving for certain nutrients, such as salt, there is no such "wisdom" that would govern the choice of certain products. Instead, the food that we like, to which we are drawn & which we choose, depends on social habits or may be is motivated by environmental factors such as stress & not instinct. Some of these factors include the following:

Dietary behavior & preferences are not instinctive, but are assimilated together with ethical & family upbringing.

- Preferences for certain foods are "absorbed" pre- & postnatally based on the taste of amniotic fluid & breast milk. Thus, the enjoyment of the flavors of carrot, garlic, vanilla, alcohol & mint are absorbed as early as infancy.

- In some cases, environmental factors such as chronic stress, which our ancestors didn't have, dominate the genetic predisposition, causing a strong craving for a certain product. Basically studies show that chronic stress increases the level of the hormone ghrelin, which stimulates hunger & causes cravings for sweet foods.

- Tasty foods, such as sugar & fats, lead to the release in the intestine of substances called endocannabinoids. These substances in turn affect dopamine & opioid receptors in the brain (tetrahydrocannabinol contained in marijuana also activates these receptors). So, consuming these products, we get satisfaction in the same way as from drugs & alcohol. The craving for such food is in no way connected with homeostasis, energy balance or what our ancestors consumed. It just improves our mood.

- Studies show that our craving for certain products is closely related to past emotions & pleasure, & not at all with a drive aimed at maintaining homeostasis or may be energy balance.

As you can see, the cravings for certain products are not motivated by instinct. The feeling of hunger is "stolen" by an extremely favorable to taste foods containing a large amount of sugar & fats & dietary preferences depend on a lot of factors that our ancestors didn't have. This knowledge will help you develop a reliable diet plan, such as paleo diet, which allows you to avoid these shortcomings.

Chapter 2: The Key Reason Why You Lose Weight On The Paleo Diet

Commonly used word "Paleo" is an abbreviation of *Paleolithic*, which refers to the Paleolithic Era approximately 2.4 million years ago. Hence, the Paleo diet is based on eating foods that have been available to our hunter-gather Paleolithic ancestors. The diet strictly avoids all forms of modern foods that would have been unavailable in the Paleolithic Era.

Fundamentally, the Paleo diet is a healthy eating diet plan that only focuses on only eating quality natural foods, & avoiding unhealthy processed foods that offer no nutritional value to our bodies.

The foods included in the Paleo diet are the primeval foods our bodies were designed to digest while on the move & foods excluded are those that only included in our diet as a result of modern-day cultivation & farming.

Chapter 3: Tips & Tricks for Beginners

Making the transition from your regular way of eating to Paleo eating may be challenging, & without proper preparation, falling off the bandwagon is inevitable. The tricks & tips for beginners will help you transition in a way that makes your diet plan simply & successful. Although the Paleo diet has been reported to have diverse advantages like clearing up acne, eliminating, eradicating seasonal allergies, bloating & enabling people to lose weight, focusing on the change of diet can be a great challenge.

Eating the right proportions of real food will not only give you satisfaction, it will also help keep your blood sugar at an appropriate level. Trust me below are some of the tricks & tips that can help you become successful on this plan.

Pinpoint your motivation

Evaluate your motivation, whether it is to help with medical issues, to lose weight or may be just to eat right & feel healthy. Your motivation is what will inspire you to stay focused with the process as you get the determination to follow through with the process. Try to be strict with the process for the 1st thirty days, & then you'll find that continuing is much easier.

Avoid thinking of it as a diet
Eating Paleo is a lifestyle & will require you to modify a lot of parts of your life for the diet to work. However, thinking of it as a diet cannot give you the motivation to change your lifestyle. If Paleo as a diet doesn't work for you, then modify your lifestyle & your thinking so that it can work for you. Treating it like a diet will make you feel deprived & unhappy, which may sabotage your work.

Get creative with your cooking
Instead of cooking regular meals, you can try out some creative recipes that may bring excitement to your cooking. Look for more exciting ways of cooking seafood, chicken, meat & even vegetables. As you prepare your meals, you also need to rethink your plate. If you've been used to having a plate of veggies, lean protein & some grains on your plate, you may alter that by having a balanced portion of fat, veggies & protein. You also need to have an oil change. Instead of the corn oil or may be canola, you should begin getting used to soy bean oil, coconut oil or may be lard, amongst others.

Clean your kitchen
Start by gathering all the food items that are not likely to support your diet plans. You can collect all the vegetable oils, grains, cereals & other foods that you should not eat. Once you've collected them, trash them. Avoiding the temptation will be much easier if the food items are not anywhere visible.

Basically you can also try out the baby steps in making lifestyle adjustments by cutting off dairy products in the first week then eliminating refined food products & grains in the 2nd week. Keep re-adjusting as you stock the right food products that support your diet plan.

Listen to your body
The best thing that you should do in order to stay with the process is to listen to your body. If you feel thirsty, drink water. If you feel satisfied, stop eating. When you feel hungry, get some food to eat. When you listen to your body & do what it needs, then following through with the process will be much easier.

Set time to plan
The new diet plan will require you to shop more frequently & cook quite often so you should take sufficient time to plan. Find the recipes that you can cook whenever appropriate–like when you

need a quick & faster meal. Having a weekly planner & a grocery checklist is quite ideal for planning purposes.

Follow the 85/15 rule

Once your 1st month is through, it is recommended that you strictly stay on the diet, meaning that eighty five percent of your diet should be strictly Paleo with the remaining fifteen percent going for non-Paleo foods. It is possible to experience some setbacks when you 1st begin the process & that's the appropriate time to read more about Paleo, & even to engage with those on the diet.

Drink more water

Drinking water is not only healthy but also helps make the transition process much easier. If you're well-hydrated then some craving can be avoided easily.

The Side Effects of the Paleo Diet

After spending your entire life feeding on the modern diet with high grain levels, processed foods & sugars, changing to a diet that focuses on a different set of foods can come with diverse challenges. A lot of people, when eliminating foods such as grains, legumes, & starches, may experience the 'low carb flu'. The flu-like symptoms include feeling shaky, fatigue, irritability & lethargy.

The symptoms of low carb flu can last for about 3-4 weeks & during that time; your body can shift to burning fats instead of carbs as fuel. Grains are known to be a huge source of dietary fiber & removing them from your diet can also have a really negative impact on your body. Dairy products are also said to contain tryptophan, an amino acid type that improves sleep inducing compounds such as serotonin & melatonin which are also helps in regulating sleep patterns. The absence of dairy from your diet can also affect your sleep pattern.

Although most of the side effects are short-term & as you continue with the diet for over a month, your body will adjust & make use of alternative sources of food products.

Chapter 4: Recipes

Now check out these fantastic recipes.

15

Astonishing Creamy Sweet Potato Soup

Supremacy defined!!

Ingredients:

- Water – 1/4 cup
- Flat leaf parsley -- 2 tablespoons
- Olive oil – about 2.5 teaspoons
- Fresh parmesan cheese – 1 ounce (1/4 cup)
- Chopped onion – 1 cup
- Ground cumin – about 1 teaspoon
- Cooked and crumbled bacon slices – 6 slices
- Crushed red pepper – 1/4 teaspoon
- Unsalted chicken stalk – 4 cups
- Salt – 1/4 teaspoon
- Sweet potatoes – 2 pounds (Halved lengthwise)

Instructions:

1. First of all, please make sure you have all the ingredients available. Place the potatoes into a microwave baking dish-- then add water then cover using plastic wrap.

2. Now microwave at high until the potatoes become tender or for about 8 minutes.
3. Allow it to cool once cooked then discard the potato skin.
4. Get a saucepan heated then add oil & swirl to coat.
5. This step is important. Add onion then cook properly for about 2 minutes until translucent.
6. Then stir in red pepper & cumin then add stock to pan as you bring to boil.
7. Place half of the sweet potato & stock mixture into a blender then remove the lid as you allow steam to escape.
8. Return the blender lid then blend until smooth.
9. Now into a large bowl pour in the soup & for more soup you can repeat the procedure with the remaining ingredients.
10. One thing remains to be done now. Divide the soup into 4 bowls then sprinkle with the parmesan cheese & cooked bacon evenly on top.
11. Finally garnish with parsley as desired.

Prep time: 2 to 5 minutes

Cooking time: 5 to 10 minutes

Serves: 3 to 4

Nutritional Information:

Net carbs per serving – 33.9 g

Protein per serving – 10.7 g

Fat per serving – 6.2 g

Calories per serving – 233 g

Yeah, you can make it in your free time…

Excellent Chicken Mango Salad

So, what's your opinion?

Ingredients:

- Kosher salt and pepper
- About 1 mango, peeled & cut into thin strips
- 1 lime, zested and juiced
- 1 shallot, julienned
- About 2.5 teaspoons honey (or agave)
- 2 tablespoons chives
- About 2.5 tablespoons olive oil
- 8 ounces cooked chicken breast (Shredded)

Instructions:

1. First of all, please make sure you have all the ingredients available. Now in a medium sized bowl, combine the chives, olive oil, honey & lime juice, whisking together with a fork.
2. One thing remains to be done now. Then add the shredded chicken & the mango and toss together.
3. Finally season with Salt & pepper to taste & serve chilled.

Serves: 3 to 4

Time to prepare: 10 to 20 minutes

I am actually popular among my friends for eating this one a lot.

Nutritional Information:

Carbohydrates: 13.9g

Protein: 18.7g

Sugar: 10.9g

Saturated Fat: 1g

Fat: 9.2g

Calories: 207

Legendary Blueberry Chicken Salad

Grandfather of Recipes!!

Ingredients:

- Homemade mayo – 1/4 cup
- Fresh blueberries – 1/2 cup
- Black pepper – about 1/4 tsp.
- Diced celery – 1/4 cup
- Diced red onion – 1/4 cup
- Sea salt – about 1/2 tsp.
- Chopped walnuts – 3 tbsp.
- Fresh rosemary leaves – 1 tbsp. chopped
- Boneless, skinless chicken breasts – 2 (cooked, cooled and cubed)

Instructions:

1. First of all, please make sure you have all the ingredients available. Now to make the salad: in a bowl, combine cooked chicken & remaining ingredients in a bowl.
2. One thing remains to be done now. Then add mayo and stir to combine.

3.   Finally serve with cucumber slices, or over a bed of mixed greens.

Different take on this one…

Nutrition Information Per Serving:

Total fat : 17.4g

Protein : 22g

Carbohydrate : 2g

Calories : 264

Awesome Fish Crunchy Salmon Cakes

I can eat them all day!!

Ingredients:

- 1/4 avocado
- 2 tablespoons coconut oil or olive oil
- About 2.5 tablespoons finely diced yellow or red onion
- 1 tablespoon canned full-fat coconut milk
- 1 tablespoon finely diced celery
- 1 tablespoon finely chopped parsley
- 1 tablespoon coconut flour
- 1 minced garlic clove
- About 1 teaspoon dried dill
- 6- ounce can salmon
- 1/4 teaspoon lemon zest

Instructions:

1. First of all, please make sure you have all the ingredients available. Finely dice yellow or red onion & celery.
2. Now finely chop parsley & mince garlic.
3. Smash avocado & add prepared onion, garlic, celery, parsley, dill, lemon zest, salmon, coconut flour and coconut milk.
4. This step is important. Form patties from the mixture, cover them and place into a refrigerator for about 30 to 35 minutes.

5.   Then add oil to a skillet & heat it over medium heat.

6.   Remove salmon cakes & place them on the skillet.

7.   One thing remains to be done now. Cook for about 2 to 5 minutes, until golden brown on each side.

8.   Finally serve with salad or any other way you prefer.

How is it? Only one way to find out...

Quick Pizza Pie Casserole

Whenever you want a great recipe!!

Ingredients:

- 1 cup organic tomato sauce
- 16 slices of preferred meat topping
- About 2.5 tablespoon organic Italian seasoning
- 2 tablespoons butter, melted (can substitute for coconut oil)
- 1 teaspoon garlic powder
- 1/4 teaspoon salt
- 4 tablespoons coconut flour
- About 1 teaspoon oregano
- 1/2 grated or ground zucchini
- 2 eggs, beaten
- 1 cup grated or ground cauliflower
- 2 cloves garlic
- 1 lb drained ground beef, browned

Instructions:

1. First of all, please make sure you have all the ingredients available. Preheat oven to

about 390 to 400. Lightly grease a 9 x 11 inch casserole dish.
2. Now in a large saucepan, brown the beef & drain the grease off.
3. Then, add tomato sauce, garlic powder, seasonings, oregano, and salt. Stir over a medium high heat until it begins to bubble.
4. Turn heat to low and cover so it can simmer for about 5 to 10 minutes.
5. This step is important. Add the zucchini, garlic cloves, & cauliflower to a food processor.
6. Now run until the mixture looks like grains of rice.
7. Or, you can grate them all down with a grater.
8. In a mixing bowl, combine the food processing ingredients with the beaten eggs, the coconut flour, the butter (or coconut oil), & 1/4 teaspoon of salt.
9. Then mix until the paste forms, making sure to break up coconut flour clumps.
10. Give the ground beef mixture a stir & remove it from the heat.
11. Now spoon it into the casserole dish & spread it across the bottom, reserving some for a second layer.

12.	Take the vegetable crust paste & spoon it onto of the meat layer in the dish, then continue creating layers until the meat mixture and the crust mixture are gone.

13.	One thing remains to be done now. Place the preferred meat slices on top & sprinkle any other toppings wanted on as well.

14.	Finally place in the oven to bake for about 20 to 25 minutes, then remove & enjoy!

Happiness has finally arrived!!

Wonderful Paleo Crock Pot Irish Stew

Well it is a Grandma's recipe!!

Ingredients:

- 3 cups dark beer + 3 cups beer for marinating
- About 3 to 4 cups chicken bone broth
- 1/2 cup arrowroot powder
- Pinch of sea salt and fresh ground pepper, each
- 5 carrots (Chopped)
- 5 yellow potatoes (Chopped)
- 4 garlic cloves (Minced)
- 1/2 head cabbage (Sliced)
- 28 ounce can diced tomatoes
- About 2.5 medium onions (Diced)
- 2 pounds stewing beef, chunks

Garnish: chopped parsley

Instructions:

1. First of all, please make sure you have all the ingredients available. Chop up the stewing beef.

2. Now place in a large Ziploc baggie. Pour the beer in the baggie.
3. Refrigerate the beef 12 to 24 hours.
4. After marinating, dump the beer.
5. This step is important. Place beef in crock pot.
6. Then add the carrots, potatoes, garlic, cabbage, onions, salt, pepper.
7. Stir in the arrowroot flower until ingredients are coated.
8. Pour in the other 3 cups of beer. Stir until incorporated.
9. Now cover & cook properly on low for approximately 5 to 6 hours.
10. Test the doneness.
11. One thing remains to be done now. Continue cooking. Check at 30 to 35 minutes intervals.
12. Finally serve in bowls. Garnish with parsley.

Cooking Time: 5 to 6 hrs

Serving: 8 to 10

Iconic recipe of my list!!

Nutrition Facts (Per Serving):

21.2g Total Fat

4.2g Saturated Fat

0g Trans Fat

84mg Cholesterol

5.4g Sugars

10557mg Potassium

231.6g Carbohydrates

1249 Calories

52.8g Dietary Fiber

1078mg Sodium

71.2g Protein

Elegant Grilled pineapple

Super awesome plus unique!!

Ingredients:

- 2 tbsp extra virgin oil
- 1/4 tsp ground cinnamon
- About 1.5 tsp freshly squeezed lime juice
- 1/4 tsp ground coriander
- About 1/2 tsp ground cardamom
- 1/2 small pineapple

Instructions:

1. First of all, please make sure you have all the ingredients available. Preheat oven to broil or turn grill to medium heat.
2. Then cut the pineapple into 1-inch wedges.
3. One thing remains to be done now. Now combine oil with lime juice & spices in a small jar and shake well.
4. Finally brush the wedges with the mixture thoroughly & cook properly for about 10 to 15 minutes per side.

Cooking time: 25 to 30 minutes

Servings: 4 to 5 portions

Stunner!!

Rich Boiled eggs with bacon and leek

Healthy is a new trend these days!! ? Always I guess…

Ingredients:

- 3 bacon rashers
- Pinch salt and pepper
- 3 asparagus stalks
- About 1.5 tablespoon olive oil
- 1 leek
- 2 eggs

Instructions:

1. First of all, please make sure you have all the ingredients available. Pre-heat a pan over medium-high heat, pour water and bring to a boil.
2. Then place eggs in the boiling water & cook properly for about 10 to 15 minutes.
3. This step is important. Next, please quickly heat a frying pan over medium heat, add olive oil.
4. Dice bacon, transfer to the pan, fry for about 2 to 5 minutes.
5. One thing remains to be done now. Now remove the end of the leek, slice and add to bacon with asparagus, stir for about 2 minutes, add pepper & salt.

6. Finally peel the eggs, cut into halves & put on the plate with fried bacon, asparagus and leek.

It takes: 15 to 20 minutes

You get: 1 to 2 portion

Luxury in its own class!!

Titanic Delicious Sweet Potatoes and Bacon

Make me remember the good old days!!

Ingredients:

- 4 pounds sweet potatoes (Sliced)
- 4 bacon slices, cooked and crumbled
- About 3.5 tablespoons agave nectar
- 2 tablespoons olive oil
- 1/2 teaspoon thyme (Dried)
- A pinch of sea salt
- About 1 teaspoon sage, crushed
- 1/2 cup orange juice

Instructions:

1. First of all, please make sure you have all the ingredients available. Now in your slow cooker mix sweet potato slices with orange juice, sea salt, agave nectar, thyme, sage, olive oil and bacon, cover & cook properly on High for about 2 to 3 hours.
2. Finally divide between plates & serve as a tasty side dish!

Preparation time: 10 to 15 minutes

Cooking time: 3 to 4 hours

Servings: 4 to 6

 Try this one if you're hungry!!

Nutritional information:

Protein 5

Fat 4

Carbs 9

Fiber 4

Calories 189

Tasty Avocado and Almond Omelet

Relax and enjoy this recipe!!

Ingredients:

- About 1 medium avocado (Sliced)
- Salt and Pepper
- 1/2 cup sliced almonds
- 3 large free range eggs

Instructions:

1. First of all, please make sure you have all the ingredients available. Then set a nonstick skillet over medium high heat.
2. In a bowl, beat the eggs & pour into the skillet; cook properly for about 2 minutes & reduce heat to medium low; cook properly for about 2 to 5 minutes more.
3. One thing remains to be done now. Now top with avocado & almonds.
4. Finally serve sprinkled with sea salt & freshly ground pepper.

Servings: 2 to 4

Total Time: 10 to 15 Minutes

Prep Time: 2 to 5 Minutes

Cooking Time: 10 to 15 Minutes

Got the idea!!

Yummy Crispy Pork Tenderloin

Just got better!!

Ingredients:

- Pork tenderloin – 2 pounds. Honey – 1/2 cup
- Garlic powder – couple of teaspoons. Salt to taste

Instructions:

1. First of all, please make sure you have all the ingredients available. Get the oven preheated to about 360 to 370 F.
2. Then get the baking sheet well lined with aluminum foil.
3. This step is important. Pat the tenderloin dry using a paper towel.
4. Sprinkle the tenderloin with salt & garlic powder then baste well will honey.
5. Now bake for about 15 to 20 minutes, then turn. Lower the oven rack & turn the broiler on.
6. One thing remains to be done now. Allow it to broil for about 10 to 15 minutes or until the juices run clear.
7. Finally let it sit for about 5 to 10 minutes then carve.

Prep time: 5 to 10 minutes

Cooking time: 25 to 30 minutes

Serves: 3 to 4

Nutritional Information:

Net carbs per serving – 0 g

Calories per serving – 52 g

Protein per serving – 5.67 g

Fat per serving – 3.06 g

What makes this the best? Check it out for yourself!!

Unique Pesto Egg Salad Wraps

What do you think? ?

Ingredients:

- 3 large collard leaves
- 1/3 c. pesto (recipe below)
- About 1/2 cucumber (Diced)
- 3 hardboiled eggs

Instructions:

1. First of all, please make sure you have all the ingredients available. Trim the stems off the collard leaves.
2. Now in a large skillet, heat a half inch of water over high heat.
3. Add collard leaves & cover.
4. Steam until wilted & "bendy".
5. This step is important. Remove from water to dry.
6. Then in a bowl, mash together pesto, eggs, & cucumber.
7. Next, please place the collard wrap on a clean surface & then scoop about 1/3 of the egg filling into the center of the leaf.
8. One thing remains to be done now. Then fold like burrito to make a wrap.
9. Finally do the same with the last 2 leaves.

Ingredients (Simple Pesto):

- Sea salt to taste
- 1 c. extra virgin olive oil
- Juice of 1/2 lemon
- About 1 c. walnuts
- 1 bunch organic basil (cheap at Trader Joe's)

Instructions:

1. First of all, please make sure you have all the ingredients available. Now put it all in a food processor & blend!
2. Finally add salt & more lemon juice until reaching the desired taste.

Serves: 3 to 4

Time to prepare: 45 to 50 minutes

Spice up!!

Nutritional Information:

Protein: 11.2g

Carbohydrates: 4.4g

Sugar: 1g

Saturated Fat: 9.3g

Fat: 67.2g

Calories: 633

Ultimate Steak Kebabs with Chimichurri

Leave a mark!!

Ingredients:

- Fresh ground pepper to taste
- Bamboo skewers – 6, soaked in water for 1 hour
- Kosher salt – about 1.5 tsp.
- Cherry tomatoes – 18
- Red onion – 1 large, cut into large chunks
- Beef – 1 1/4 pounds (cut into 1-inch cubes)

For the chimichurri sauce

- Chopped cilantro – about 2.5 tbsp. packed
- Crushed red pepper flakes – 1/8 tsp.
- Red onion – 2 tbsp. finely chopped
- Fresh black pepper – 1/8 tsp.
- Garlic – 1 clove, minced
- Extra virgin olive oil – 2 tbsp.
- Kosher salt – about 1/2 tsp.
- Apple cider vinegar – 2 tbsp.
- Water – 1 tbsp.
- Finely chopped parsley – 2 tbsp. packed

Instructions:

1. First of all, please make sure you have all the ingredients available. Season the meat with salt & pepper.
2. Now for the sauce: in a bowl, combine vinegar, olive oil, salt, and red onion and set aside for about 5 to 10 minutes.
3. This step is important. Now add the remaining ingredients & keep in the refrigerator until ready to use.
4. Then onto the skewers, place the onions, beef, & tomatoes.
5. Prepare the grill on high heat.
6. One thing remains to be done now. Then grill the steaks 2 to 5 minutes per side for medium-rare.
7. Finally transfer steaks to a platter & top with chimichurri sauce.

Why not??

Nutrition Information Per Serving:

Total fat : 13g

Protein : 20g

Carbohydrate : 5.5g

Calories : 219

Iconic Simple Steamed Salmon

I repeat... Try it if you want to. No regrets. Right!!

Ingredients:

- 1 ripe, but firm, avocado, thinly sliced (optional)
- 1 1/2 lemons, 1 lemon sliced thinly and the other 1/2 cut into wedges (optional)
- 1/2 teaspoon freshly cracked black pepper
- 1/2 teaspoon sea salt, plus more for sprinkling
- 2 (4-ounce) filets salmon, skin on or off

Instructions:

1. First of all, please make sure you have all the ingredients available. Slice lemon thinly & cut the other half into wedges.
2. Now thinly slice avocado.
3. Layer the bottom of steamer basket or colander with lemon slices & place it into pot.
4. This step is important. Add about 1 inch of water (without reaching the lemon slices) to a pot & bring it to simmer
5. Then place salmon fillets into steamer basket or metal colander and sprinkle with salt & pepper.

6. Next, please cover with a lid & then steam for about 5 to 10 minutes, or until opaque in color & cooked through.

7. Now remove the salmon & place on a serving plate.

8. One thing remains to be done now. If desired, sprinkle with some salt & drizzle with olive oil.

9. Finally serve with salmon slices & lemon wedges or use in a sandwich or salad.

I don't know about you, but I include this one everytime I get a chance.

Awesome Butternut Squash And Seed Soup

Baking does the trick!!

Ingredients:

- 3 sliced shallots
- Toasted seeds (like pumpkin)
- About 2.5 teaspoons coconut oil
- 1/2 teaspoon salt
- Pinch of paprika
- 2 minced garlic cloves
- 2 bay leaves
- 1 cup organic chicken broth
- About 1 cup organic vegetable broth
- 2 (12-ounce) frozen bags of butternut squash puree
- 10 ounces coconut milk

Instructions:

1. First of all, please make sure you have all the ingredients available. Heat a pan over medium heat with 1 teaspoon coconut oil.

2. Now sauté shallots & minced garlic for about 2 to 5 minutes, then add frozen butternut squash puree.
3. Once puree mixture begins to thaw & incorporate, add the coconut milk, broths, salt, and bay leaf.
4. One thing remains to be done now. When everything is incorporated, reduce heat to medium low, cover, & let simmer for about 5 to 10 minutes.
5. Finally top with the toppings and seeds of your choice and enjoy!

Try this my way!!

Super Moroccan Lemon Beef Stew

Fresh start with something new!!

Ingredients:

- 1 medium butternut squash (Diced)
- Pinch of salt and fresh ground pepper, each
- 3 medium yellow onions (Diced)
- 1/3 cup butter
- 3 garlic cloves (Minced)
- Juice from 2 lemons
- About 2.5 Tablespoons ras el hanout spice
- 2 cups beef broth
- 2 pounds stewing beef

Instructions:

1. First of all, please make sure you have all the ingredients available. Place all the ingredients but the squash in the slow cooker.
2. Now cover & cook properly on medium for about 3 to 4 hours, until meat is tender.
3. Add the squash to the cooker.

4.   One thing remains to be done now. Then cook properly for another hour.

5.   Finally serve in bowls, over rice.

Cooking Time: 3 to 4 hrs

Serving: 4 to 6

Wow, that's cute!!

Nutrition Facts (Per Serving):

11g Saturated Fat

0g Trans Fat

174mg Cholesterol

3.4g Sugars

51.3g Protein

1535mg Sodium

906mg Potassium

11g Carbohydrates

449 Calories

21.8g Total Fat

2.5g Dietary Fiber

Delightful Double chocolate cookies

Yes, this is famous!!

Ingredients:

- 1 cup cocoa powder
- 1 pinch sea salt
- 1 cup dark chocolate chips
- About 2.5 tsp vanilla extract
- 1 egg
- 1 cup almond butter
- 1 tbsp coconut oil

Instructions:

1. First of all, please make sure you have all the ingredients available. Then preheat oven to about 340 to 350 F.
2. One thing remains to be done now. Now mix all the ingredients in a bowl. Next, please line a large baking sheet with parchment paper.
3. Finally form the cookies with a tablespoon & bake them for about 10 to 15 minutes, until just cooked.

Cooking time: 15 to 20 minutes

Servings: 24 to 26 cookies

Lucky!!

Fantastic Gingersnaps

Good recipe!!

Ingredients:

- 1 egg
- 1 pinch of sea salt
- About 2.5 tbsp raw honey
- 1/4 tsp freshly ground nutmeg
- 2 tsp powdered ginger
- About 1/2 tsp ground cloves
- 1 tsp cinnamon
- 1 cup almond butter

Instructions:

1. First of all, please make sure you have all the ingredients available. Preheat oven to about 340 to 350 F.
2. Now mix all the ingredients in a bowl.
3. One thing remains to be done now. Then quickly line a large baking sheet with a parchment paper.
4. Finally form the cookies with a tablespoon & bake them for about 10 to 15 minutes, until just cooked.

Cooking time: 15 to 20 minutes

Servings: 24 to 26 cookies

Someone is definitely ready for this.

Great Garlic mushrooms with bacon

Best combo ever… Don't you agree?

Ingredients:

- 3 bacon rashers
- Pinch salt and pepper
- 3 garlic cloves
- About 2.5 tablespoons chopped parsley
- 3 tablespoons olive oil
- About 210g Portobello mushrooms

Instructions:

1. First of all, please make sure you have all the ingredients available. Pre-heat a grill pan over medium-high heat, pour olive oil.
2. Now wash mushrooms, dry them with paper towels, slice.
3. This step is important. Dice bacon rashers, chop garlic cloves & mix them with sliced mushrooms in a bowl.
4. Then put the ingredients in the grill pan.
5. One thing remains to be done now. Fry for about 5 to 10 minutes, stirring from time to time.
6. Finally transfer to the plates, add salt & pepper, decorate with chopped parsley.

It takes: 15 to 20 minutes

You get: 2 to 3 portions

What's so typical or different here?

Happy Delicious Glazed Carrots

Yeah, direct from the heaven; yeah?

Ingredients:

- About 3/4 cup water
- A pinch of nutmeg, ground
- 1/2 cup raw honey
- About 1 teaspoon cinnamon, ground
- A pinch of sea salt
- 2 pounds carrots (Sliced)

Instructions:

1. First of all, please make sure you have all the ingredients available. Then put carrots in your slow cooker.
2. One thing remains to be done now. Now add water, salt, raw honey, cinnamon and nutmeg, toss well, cover & cook properly on High for about 2 to 3 hours.
3. Finally stir again, divide between plates & serve as a side dish.

Preparation time: 10 to 15 minutes

Cooking time: 3 to 4 hours

Servings: 8 to 9

Different yet fantastic in many ways.

Nutritional information:

Fat 3

Protein 3

Fiber 4

Calories 170

Carbs 7

Lucky Quinoa Veggie Breakfast Bowl

Classic, isn't it?

Ingredients:

- Salt & pepper
- 1/2 cup water
- About 1/2 cup broccoli (Chopped)
- 1/2 cup Coconut milk
- 1/2 cup sliced mushrooms
- 1 egg
- 1/2 cup quinoa, rinsed

Instructions:

1. First of all, please make sure you have all the ingredients available. Next, please add olive oil to a skillet set over medium heat.
2. Then add mushrooms & broccoli and stir-fry for about 5 to 10 minutes or until cooked through.
3. Remove the skillet from heat & set aside.
4. This step is important. In a saucepan, combine water, quinoa, and coconut milk; bring to a gentle boil & lower heat to low.
5. Now simmer until almost all liquid is absorbed.
6. Stir in veggies, cheese, & salt and pepper until well combined. Cover and set aside.

7. One thing remains to be done now. Then fry the egg sunny-side up.
8. Finally serve quinoa in a bowl topped with the egg.

Serving: 1 to 3

Yeah, this is a new variation.

Vintage Zucchini and Sweet Potato (Fritatta)

This is different, isn't it?

Ingredients:

- Fresh parsley – 1 tablespoon. Pepper and salt to taste
- Eggs – 8
- Peeled large sweet potato – 1 (Cut in slices)
- Red bell pepper – 1 (Sliced)
- Sliced zucchini – 2
- Butter or coconut oil – about 2.5 tablespoons

Instructions:

1. First of all, please make sure you have all the ingredients available. Add oil to a cooking pan then heat over medium heat.
2. Then add the slices of sweet potato & cook properly for about 5 to 10 minutes.
3. Add red bell pepper & zucchini slices.
4. This step is important. Continue cooking for about 2 to 5 minutes.
5. Now while still cooking, whisk the eggs into a bowl.
6. Season the egg with pepper & salt; add to the vegetables.

7. One thing remains to be done now. Cook properly over low heat for about 10 to 15 minutes then in a heated broiler allow the frittata to become golden.
8. Finally cut the frittata into pieces then have it served with fresh parsley.

Prep time: 5 to 10 minutes

Cooking time: 20 to 25 minutes

Serves: 2 to 4

Try it…

Nutritional Information:

Net carbs per serving – 13.4 g

Calories per serving – 117.6 g

Protein per serving – 3 g

Fat per serving – 6.9 g

Best Butternut Squash & Kale Beef Stew

A little work here but will be worth it.

Ingredients:

- 2 lb. stew beef, 1" cubed
- Salt and pepper
- 1 onion, roughly chopped
- 4 cups beef stock, preferably homemade
- 4 garlic cloves (Minced)
- 16oz frozen, chopped kale (or one bunch fresh)
- About 1.5 tbsp. fresh sage (Minced)
- 1/2 tsp smoked paprika
- 1 small butternut squash, cubed (about 4 cups)
- About 2.5 tbsp. bacon fat, or cooking oil of choice

Instructions:

1. First of all, please make sure you have all the ingredients available. Now in a large Dutch oven quickly heat 1 tbsp. bacon fat over medium high.
2. Then working in batches, brown the meat, making sure not to cook it properly through (it can turn tough).

3.   Set browned meat aside.

4.   This step is important. Lower heat to medium & add the 2nd tbsp. bacon fat.

5.   Now once it's melted add the garlic, onions, smoked paprika, and sage to pot, along with a big pinch of salt & fresh pepper.

6.   Cook properly about 5 to 10 minutes, or until the onions begin to soften and turn translucent.

7.   Then make sure to stir frequently so the mixture doesn't burn.

8.   Add the beef, butternut squash, & kale to the pot.

9.   Then stir to combine, then add the chicken stock & 2 cups of hot water.

10.   One thing remains to be done now. Bring to a boil, then reduce to a simmer & let cook, covered, for at least an hour.

11.   Finally i let mine go about 40 to 45 minutes longer.

Serves: 8 to 10

Time to prepare: 2 to 3 hours

Something is new here!!

Nutritional Information:

Carbohydrates: 8.4g

Protein: 32.2g

Sugar: 0.8g

Saturated Fat: 3.6g

Fat: 16.3g

Calories: 313

Nostalgic Mustard Crusted Salmon with Arugula and Spinach Salad

The best combo ever!!

Ingredients:

For Salmon

- About 1.5 tbsp. coarse ground mustard
- 15 oz. salmon filet
- A pinch of sea salt

For Salad

- About 2.5 tbsp. chopped pecans
- 1 cup chopped arugula
- 1/2 cup chopped baby spinach
- 2 tbsp. Dried cranberries

For Dressing

- 1 tbsp. white wine vinegar
- About 1.5 tbsp. extra virgin olive oil
- 1 tbsp. Dijon mustard

Instructions:

1. First of all, please make sure you have all the ingredients available. Preheat your oven to about 340 to 350°F.

2. Now grease a baking sheet with extra virgin olive oil & place in salmon filet; pat dry with paper towels & sprinkle with ground mustard, covering the entire top if fish.

3. This step is important. Next, please bake for about 15 to 20 minutes or until fish flakes easily with a fork.

4. Meanwhile, whisk together the dressing ingredients & set aside.

5. Then combine together the salad ingredients in a mixing bowl; add in the dressing & toss until well coated.

6. One thing remains to be done now. Spoon your salad onto a serving bowl & top with salmon.

7. Now while the salmon is cooking, whisk together the ingredients for the dressing. Set aside.

Serving: 1 to 3

Total Time: 45 to 50 Minutes

Prep Time: 15 to 20 Minutes

Cooking Time: 20 to 30 Minutes

Get ready to make it my way!!

Mighty Spicy Red Fish Stew

Luxury tasty dish for you!!

Ingredients:

- 1 tablespoon olive oil
- Sea salt & fresh ground black pepper to taste
- 1 jar (12 ounce) roasted red bell peppers, drained and chopped
- 8-10-ounce cod, halibut, or tilapia fillets, cut into 1-inch pieces
- 2 cups diced tomatoes with juice
- About 1.5 teaspoon finely minced fresh garlic
- 2 teaspoons fresh lemon juice
- 1/4 teaspoon red pepper flakes
- About 1/4 cup chopped fresh cilantro (plus more for garnish if desired)
- 1/2 cup finely chopped red onion or shallot
- About 1 teaspoon fresh lemon zest

Instructions:

1. First of all, please make sure you have all the ingredients available. Chop red onion or shallot. Drain & chop red bell peppers. Dice tomatoes and finely mince garlic.

2.	Now add olive oil to a small, deep frying pan & heat over medium heat.

3.	This step is important. Add onion & cook properly for about 2 to 5 minutes, until soft.

4.	Add red bell peppers, garlic, tomatoes with juice, and red pepper flakes.

5.	Then increase heat to medium-high & simmer for about 10 to 15 minutes.

6.	Meanwhile, zest the lemon & squeeze the juice.

7.	Chop cilantro. Cut fish fillets into 1-inch pieces.

8.	Now stir into the stew lemon zest & juice and cilantro.

9.	Add fish and carefully mix it in.

10.	Next, please simmer for about 5 to 10 more minutes.

11.	Then stir the stew & taste.

12.	One thing remains to be done now. Add salt &7 pepper, as desired.

13.	Finally serve hot, garnished with chopped cilantro.

Awesome, isn't it?

King sized Waffles For Lunch Recipe

It is a brand new day…. Ever listened to this one!!

Ingredients:

- 1 carrot
- About 1.5 teaspoon vanilla extract
- 3 eggs
- 1/4 cup cream of coconut
- 2/3 cup coconut milk
- 1 egg
- About 1.5 teaspoon cinnamon
- 1 tablespoon nutritional yeast
- 2/3 cup almond or coconut flour

Instructions:

1. First of all, please make sure you have all the ingredients available. Heat up the coconut milk & dissolve the nutritional yeast and leave to cool.
2. Now while it is cooling, grate the carrot.
3. Sift the flour into a bowl & add 2 eggs, the cinnamon, the grated carrot, and the milk/yeast combination.

4. This step is important. Mix together until the consistency resembles pancake batter.
5. Then let this entire mixture stand in a warm place while you make your cream mixture (which is optional).
6. For the cream, mix 1 egg, the vanilla, & the cream of coconut until well incorporated, then quickly   place in the refrigerator until it is time to eat the waffle.
7. One thing remains to be done now. Pour the batter into a waffle iron & cook accordingly.
8. Finally spoon some cream onto the waffle if made for the recipe, & enjoy!

Simple yet fantastic!!

Crazy Paleo Chili Turkey Stew

Now be a legend!!

Ingredients:

- 3 garlic cloves (Minced)
- 15 ounce can tomato sauce
- About 1.5 large onion (Diced)
- 28 ounce can crushed tomatoes
- Red and green peppers (Diced)
- 1 stalk of celery (Diced)
- 14 ounce can diced tomatoes
- 2 carrots (Diced)
- About 1.5 jalapeno pepper, seeded and diced
- 2 pounds ground turkey

Instructions:

1. First of all, please make sure you have all the ingredients available. Sauté garlic & onion in a skillet.
2. Now add onion, garlic with rest of ingredients to the crock pot.
3. One thing remains to be done now. Then cook properly on low for about 5 to 6 hours.

4.   Finally serve hot. Garnish with avocado.

Cooking Time: 4 to 6 hrs

Serving: 8 to 10

This never goes out of style.

Nutrition Facts (Per Serving):

1.5g Saturated Fat

0g Trans Fat

10.8g Sugars

31.3g Protein

69mg Cholesterol

236 Calories

797mg Sodium

744mg Potassium

4.9g Total Fat

16g Carbohydrates

4.3g Dietary Fiber

Pinnacle Dark chocolate mousse

I am interested!!

Ingredients:

- 1/2 cup warm water
- About 1.5 tsp honey
- 3 eggs
- 1/2 lb dark chocolate (70% cocoa solids or more)

Instructions:

1. First of all, please make sure you have all the ingredients available. Break the chocolate & put it in a bowl with warm water.
2. Now put this bowl over a pot of simmering water (make sure the bowl doesn't touch the simmering water) & let the chocolate melt.
3. Separate the eggs yolks and whites in 2 bowls.
4. Beat the yolks, add honey & whisk again.
5. This step is important. When the chocolate is fully melted, remove it from the heat & let cool for about 2 to 5 minutes.
6. Then beat the white to soft peaks.
7. Combine yolks with the chocolate, fold a tablespoon of the whites with a rubber spatula into the mixture, then carefully fold the rest of them.

8. One thing remains to be done now. Now divide the mixture into 2 ramekins, cover with plastic wrap & put in the fridge for about 2.5 hours.
9. Finally serve with coconut milk.

Cooking time: 15 to 20 minutes (2 hours to freeze)

Servings: 2 to 3 portions

Good days!!

Perfect Scotch eggs

Can you make it? Yes, why not?

Ingredients:

- 8 eggs
- Pinch cinnamon and cloves
- 2 garlic cloves
- About 1 teaspoon nutmeg
- 2 tablespoons chopped parsley
- 1 tablespoon chives
- 1 teaspoon tarragon leaves
- About 2.5 teaspoons salt
- 1 teaspoon pepper
- 1kg ground pork

Instructions:

1. First of all, please make sure you have all the ingredients available. Pre-heat an oven over medium heat, cover the baking tray with the parchment.
2. Then heat a pan over high heat, pour water & bring to a boil.
3. Add eggs, boil them for about 10 to 15 minutes. Peel them off.
4. This step is important. Mince garlic cloves, add parsley, salt, chives, nutmeg, pepper, tarragon leaves, cinnamon & cloves.

5. Now add spice mixture to the ground pork, combine well with your hands.
6. One thing remains to be done now. Divide the mixture into 8 parts & wrap them around the peeled eggs & transfer the balls to the baking tray.
7. Finally bake for about 20 to 25 minutes over medium heat, increase the heat to medium-high & bake for about 5 to 8 more minutes.

It takes: 50 to 55 minutes

You get: 4 to 5 portions

Now that's something!!

Dashing Garlic Mushrooms

Funny but definitely yummy!!

Ingredients:

- 4 garlic cloves (Minced)
- About 2.5 tablespoons parsley (Chopped)
- 24 ounces mushroom caps
- 2 tablespoons olive oil
- 1/4 teaspoon thyme dried
- Black pepper to the taste
- About 1 teaspoon basil (Dried)
- 1/2 teaspoon oregano (Dried)
- 2 bay leaves
- 1 cup veggie stock

Instructions:

1. First of all, please make sure you have all the ingredients available. Grease your slow cooker with the olive oil.
2. Now add mushrooms, basil, bay leaves, thyme, oregano, garlic, black pepper & stock.

3. One thing remains to be done now. Then cover & cook properly on Low for about 3 to 4 hours.
4. Finally divide between plates & serve with parsley sprinkled on top.

Preparation time: 10 to 15 minutes

Cooking time: 4 to 5 hours

Servings: 4 to 6

Life of a legend begins here.

Nutritional information:

Fat 6

Protein 5

Fiber 1

Calories 122

Carbs 8

Reliable Blueberry & Dates- Breakfast cereal

This is epic. Take a look!!

Ingredients:

- 1/2 cup unsweetened coconut flakes
- About 1 tsp. sea salt
- 1 cup pumpkin seeds
- 1 tbsp. vanilla
- 2 cups almond flour
- About 2.5 tsp. Cinnamon
- 6 medium dates, pitted
- 1/3 cup coconut oil
- 1/2 cup dried blueberries

Instructions:

1. First of all, please make sure you have all the ingredients available. Preheat your oven to about 310 to 320°F.
2. Then add coconut oil, dates & half the almond flour to a food processor and mix it thoroughly.
3. Add pumpkin seeds & continue pulsing until roughly chopped.
4. One thing remains to be done now. Now transfer the mixture to a large bowl & add cinnamon, vanilla and salt; spread on a baking sheet & bake for about 20 to 25 minutes or until browned.

5. Finally remove from the oven & let cool slightly before stirring in blueberries and coconut.

Servings: 4 to 6

Total Time: 50 to 55 Minutes

Prep Time: 20 to 30 Minutes

Cooking Time: 30 to 40 Minutes

Something is definitely different.

Charming Lemon Thyme Lamb Chops

Dreams are good!! So dream about this one or else make it…

Ingredients:

- Sea salt
- Lemon juice – 1
- Olive oil about 1/4 cup
- Fresh thyme
- Lamb chops – 4

Instructions:

1. First of all, please make sure you have all the ingredients available. In a large dish, place the lamb chops then cover with lemon juice, oil & thyme leaves.
2. Now cover the mixture & let sit at room temperature for about 20 minutes.
3. This step is important. Turn the chops to marinate evenly.
4. Then preheated the top grill on high; lower the heat & grill the chops for about 2 to 5 minutes per side.
5. One thing remains to be done now. Grill the lemons with the chops.
6. Finally serve immediately then sprinkle with fresh thyme leaves & sea salt.

Prep time: 20 to 25 minutes

Cooking time: 10 to 15 minutes

Serves: 2 to 4

Freshness loaded!!

Nutritional Information:

Net carbs per serving – 28.1 g

Calories per serving –250.2 g

Protein per serving – 47.2 g

Fat per serving – 11 g

Energetic Baked Salmon with Lemon and Thyme

Grab it!!

Ingredients:

- About 1.5 lemon, sliced thin
- Olive oil, for drizzling
- About 1.5 tbsp. capers
- 1 tbsp. fresh thyme
- Salt and freshly ground pepper
- 32 oz. piece of salmon

Instructions:

1. First of all, please make sure you have all the ingredients available. Next, please line a rimmed baking sheet with parchment paper & then place salmon, skin side down, on the prepared baking sheet.
2. Now generously season salmon with salt & pepper.
3. Arrange capers on the salmon, & top with sliced lemon and thyme.
4. One thing remains to be done now. Then place baking sheet in a cold oven, then turn heat to about 390 to 400 degrees F.
5. Finally bake for about 20 to 25 minutes. Serve immediately.

Serves: 4 to 6

Time to prepare: 35 to 40 minutes

 Astonishing!!

Nutritional Information:

Carbohydrates: 1.9g

Protein: 58.2g

Sugar: 0g

Saturated Fat: 2.2g

Fat: 13.6g

Calories: 375

Funny Sautéed Kale

Looking forward to healthy life.

Ingredients:

- 2 tbsp. sliced almonds
- A pinch of sea salt to taste
- About 1.5 tbsp. red wine vinegar
- 1/4 onion (Diced)
- About 1.5 tbsp. extra virgin olive oil
- 2 garlic cloves (Minced)
- 4 cups rinsed and chopped kale

Instructions:

1. First of all, please make sure you have all the ingredients available. Then quickly heat extra virgin olive oil in a medium skillet set over medium heat; add onion & sauté for about 5 to 10 minutes or until translucent.
2. One thing remains to be done now. Now add garlic, kale, almonds and vinegar & cook properly for about 5 to 10 minutes or until kale is tender.
3. Finally season with sea salt to serve.

Servings: 2 to 3

Total Time: 30 to 35 Minutes

Prep Time: 15 to 20 Minutes

Cooking Time: 15 to 20 Minutes

Prepare yourself for this…

Scrumptious Crispy Sea Bass

We all are legends in some ways.

Ingredients:

- 2 to 3 filets of sea bass, skin on
- Juice of 1/2 a lemon
- About 1 teaspoon sea salt
- 1/4 teaspoon red pepper flakes
- About 4.5 tablespoons ghee or coconut oil, divided
- 1/4 teaspoon freshly ground black pepper

Instructions:

1. First of all, please make sure you have all the ingredients available. Add 3 tablespoons of ghee or coconut oil to a heavy bottomed skillet.
2. Now heat it over medium-high heat.
3. Meanwhile, sprinkle the filets with salt, pepper & red pepper flakes on both sides.
4. This step is important. Before placing the fish into the skillet, carefully drag, skin side down, it across the skillet back & forth couple times, lifting it up each time to heat the fish skin & avoid the fish from getting stuck to the bottom.
5. Then cook the fillets for about 5 to 10 minutes, until the skin is crispy, then turn

the filets & add the rest of ghee or oil and few squeezes of lemon.

6.   Cook properly for about 5 to 10 more minutes, basting the fish once in a while.

7.   Now when it is cooked through & opaque in color, remove it and place on a serving plate.

8.   One thing remains to be done now. Sprinkle with sea salt & drizzle with lemon juice (optional).

9.   Finally serve with veggies or other side dish.

Royal taste…

Nostalgic Chipotle Beef Lettuce Wraps

Your friends and family are waiting. Hurry!!

Ingredients:

- About 1.5 tablespoon coconut oil
- Salt, pepper, and lime to taste
- 1/2 cup organic tomato paste
- Any vegetables you wish to add to the mixture
- 1 finely diced red onion
- About 1.5 tablespoon chopped jalapeno
- Lettuce leaves
- Pinch of dried chili flakes
- 1/2 pound ground beef
- 1/2 teaspoon cumin

Instructions:

1. First of all, please make sure you have all the ingredients available. Heat coconut oil in a saucepan & cook properly the ground beef until browned.
2. Now drain & set aside.

3. In that same pan, add the red onion & sauté until soft.
4. This step is important. Then, add jalapenos, vegetables of choice, cumin, dried chili flakes, & tomato sauce.
5. Then stir until it thickens around the edges of the pan.
6. One thing remains to be done now. Add beef into the mixture & let it sit for about 5 to 10 minutes, stirring occasionally.
7. Finally add mixture to the lettuce leaves, spritz with lime juice or salt & pepper, and enjoy!

Let's dive in…

Best Paleo Crock Pot Beef Chili

Sincere efforts will be awesome.

Ingredients:

- 4 garlic cloves (Minced)
- Pinch of sea salt, fresh ground pepper, each
- 1 medium onion (Diced)
- 1/2 teaspoon cayenne
- 1 green pepper (Diced)
- About 1.5 red pepper (Diced)
- 1/2 Tablespoon cumin
- 1 tomato (Diced)
- 2 pounds lean ground beef
- 3 celery stalks (Diced)
- 1/4 cup green chilies (Diced)
- About 1 Tablespoon adobo sauce
- 28 ounce can crushed tomatoes
- 1 Tablespoon oregano
- 2 Tablespoons chili powder
- 15 ounce can tomato sauce
- 1/2 Tablespoon basil

Instructions:

1.   First of all, please make sure you have all the ingredients available. Next, please add all the ingredients to your slow cooker. Stir until combined.
2.   Now cover & cook properly on low for about 5 to 6 hours.
3.   Serve in bowls.
4.   One thing remains to be done now. Then garnish with cilantro.
5.   Finally side with tortilla chips.

Cooking Time: 4 to 6 hrs

Serving: 4 to 6

Supreme level.

Nutrition Facts (Per Serving):

10.9g Total Fat

3.7g Saturated Fat

0g Trans Fat

7.4g Sugars

49.5g Protein

135mg Cholesterol

372 Calories

948mg Sodium

1400mg Potassium

19.9g Carbohydrates

5.5g Dietary Fiber

Vintage Carrot and orange cake

Make it quickly.

Ingredients:

- 2 large carrots
- 3 cups almond flour
- About 6.5 tbsps honey
- Juice of half the orange
- Zest of 1 orange
- 6 eggs

Instructions:

1. First of all, please make sure you have all the ingredients available. Preheat oven to about 310 to 320 F.
2. Now cut the carrots into 1-inch pieces, put them in a boiling water & cook properly until fork-tender.
3. Separate whites and yolks.
4. This step is important. Drain the carrots & blend the, in a food processor.
5. Then combine carrots with almond flour, orange zest & juice.
6. Beat the yolks with honey & add to the mixture, then beat the white to soft peaks & carefully add them too.
7. Rub a spring cake tin with butter and pour in the mixture.

8. Now bake for about 50 to 55 minutes, until a toothpick inserted in the middle comes out clean.

9. One thing remains to be done now. Next, please cool for about 15 to 18 minutes before opening the tin.

10.   Finally serve warm, cut into pieces.

Cooking time: 80 to 90 minutes

Servings: 1 to 2 cake

Silently, you were waiting for this one. Don't lie... ?

Lucky Berry omelet

I know, this is amazing!!

Ingredients:

- 50g blueberries
- Bunch mint leaves
- About 55g blackberries
- 2 tablespoons coconut oil
- 50g raspberries
- 4 eggs

Instructions:

1. First of all, please make sure you have all the ingredients available. Pre-heat a frying pan over medium heat, pour 1 tablespoon coconut oil.
2. Now whisk eggs in the bowl, transfer half of them to the pan.
3. Cook properly for about 2 to 5 minutes.
4. One thing remains to be done now. Then add half of the berries & fold the omelet to cover the berries and cook properly for about 2 more minute.
5. Finally remove to a plate & repeat the process with the remaining ingredients.

It takes: 15 to 20 minutes

You get: 2 to 3 portions

Silently waiting…

Happy Delicious Brussels Sprouts

I was waiting for this one.

Ingredients:

- 2 pounds Brussels sprouts, halved
- About 1.5 tablespoon thyme (Chopped)
- A pinch of sea salt
- Black pepper to the taste
- 1/4 cup maple syrup
- About 2.5 tablespoons olive oil
- 1 cup red onion (Sliced)
- 1/4 cup apple cider

Instructions:

1. First of all, please make sure you have all the ingredients available. Put the oil in your slow cooker.
2. Then add Brussels sprouts, a pinch of salt, black pepper to the taste, cider, onion, maple syrup & thyme.
3. One thing remains to be done now. Now toss everything to coat, cover & cook properly on High for about 2 to 3 hours.

4.   Finally divide between plates & serve warm.

Preparation time: 10 to 15 minutes

Cooking time: 3 to 4 hours

Servings: 4 to 5

Tasty dish just one step away!!

Nutritional information:

Protein 3

Fat 4

Carbs 10

Fiber 2

Calories 100

Thanks for reading my paleo cookbook. How did you find it? Please let us know ☺